# Cocaine

# Table of Contents

**Cocaine**

What is cocaine?

What is the scope of cocaine use in the United States?

How is cocaine used?

How does cocaine produce its effects?

What are some ways that cocaine changes the brain?

What are the short-term effects of cocaine use?

What are the long-term effects of cocaine use?

Why are cocaine users at risk for contracting HIV/AIDS and hepatitis?

What are the effects of maternal cocaine use?

How is cocaine addiction treated?

How is cutting-edge science helping us better understand addiction?

References

Where can I get further information about cocaine?

# What is cocaine?

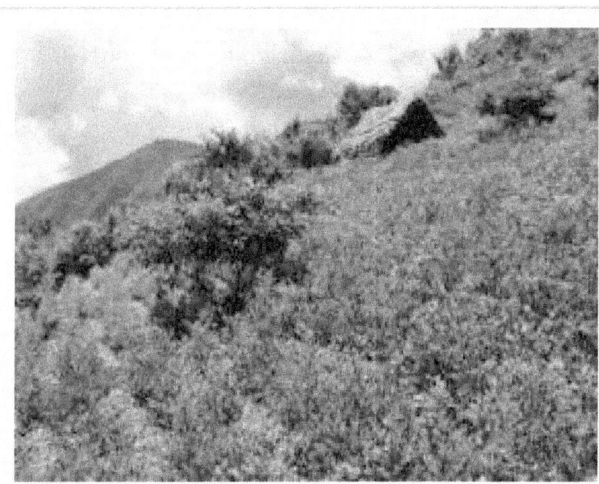

Photo by ©iStock.com/Rafal Cichawa

Cocaine is a powerfully addictive stimulant drug. For thousands of years, people in South America have chewed and ingested coca leaves (*Erythroxylon coca*), the source of cocaine, for their stimulant effects.[1,2] The purified chemical, cocaine hydrochloride, was isolated from the plant more than 100 years ago. In the early 1900s, purified cocaine was the main active ingredient in many tonics and elixirs developed to treat a wide variety of illnesses and was even an ingredient in the early formulations of Coca-Cola®. Before the development of synthetic local anesthetic, surgeons used cocaine to block pain.[1] However, research has since shown that cocaine is a powerfully addictive substance that can alter brain structure and function if used repeatedly.

Today, cocaine is a Schedule II drug, which means that it has high potential for abuse but can be administered by a doctor for legitimate medical uses, such as local anesthesia for some eye, ear, and throat surgeries. As a street drug, cocaine appears as a fine, white, crystalline powder and is also known as *Coke, C, Snow, Powder,* or *Blow*. Street dealers often dilute (or "cut") it with non-psychoactive substances such as cornstarch, talcum powder, flour, or baking soda to increase their profits. They may also adulterate cocaine with other drugs like procaine (a chemically related local anesthetic) or amphetamine (another psychoactive stimulant).[2,3] Some users combine cocaine with heroin—called a *Speedball*.[2]

People abuse two chemical forms of cocaine: the water-soluble hydrochloride salt and the water-insoluble cocaine base (or freebase). Users inject or snort the hydrochloride salt, which is a powder. The base form of cocaine is created by processing the drug with ammonia or sodium bicarbonate (baking soda) and water, then heating it to remove the hydrochloride to produce a smokable substance. The term *crack*, which is the street name given to freebase cocaine, refers to the crackling sound heard when the mixture is smoked.[2]

# What is the scope of cocaine use in the United States?

According to the National Survey on Drug Use and Health (NSDUH), cocaine use has remained relatively stable since 2009. In 2014, there were an estimated 1.5 million current (past-month) cocaine users aged 12 or older (0.6 percent of the population). Adults aged 18 to 25 years have a higher rate of current cocaine use than any other age group, with 1.4 percent of young adults reporting past-month cocaine use.[4]

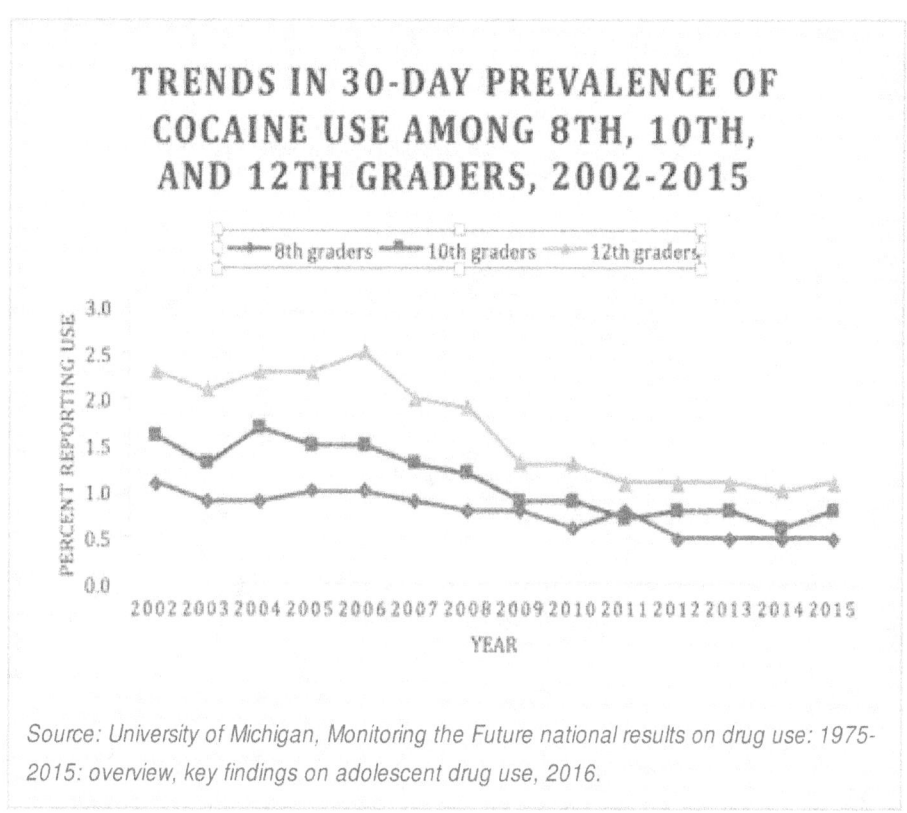

Source: University of Michigan, Monitoring the Future national results on drug use: 1975-2015: overview, key findings on adolescent drug use, 2016.

The 2015 Monitoring the Future survey, which annually surveys teen attitudes and drug use, reports a significant decline in 30-day prevalence of powder cocaine use among 8th, 10th, and 12th graders from peak use in the late 1990s. In 2014, 1.1 percent of 12th graders and only 0.8 percent of 10th and half a percent of 8th graders reported using cocaine in the past month.[5]

Repeated cocaine use can produce addiction and other adverse health consequences. In 2014, according to the NSDUH, about 913,000 Americans met the *Diagnostic and Statistical Manual of Mental Disorders* criteria for dependence or abuse of cocaine (in any form) during the past 12 months. Further, data from the 2011 Drug Abuse Warning Network (DAWN) report showed that cocaine was involved in 505,224 of the nearly 1.3 million visits to emergency departments for drug misuse or abuse. This translates to over one in three drug misuse or abuse-related emergency department visits (40 percent) that involved cocaine.[6]

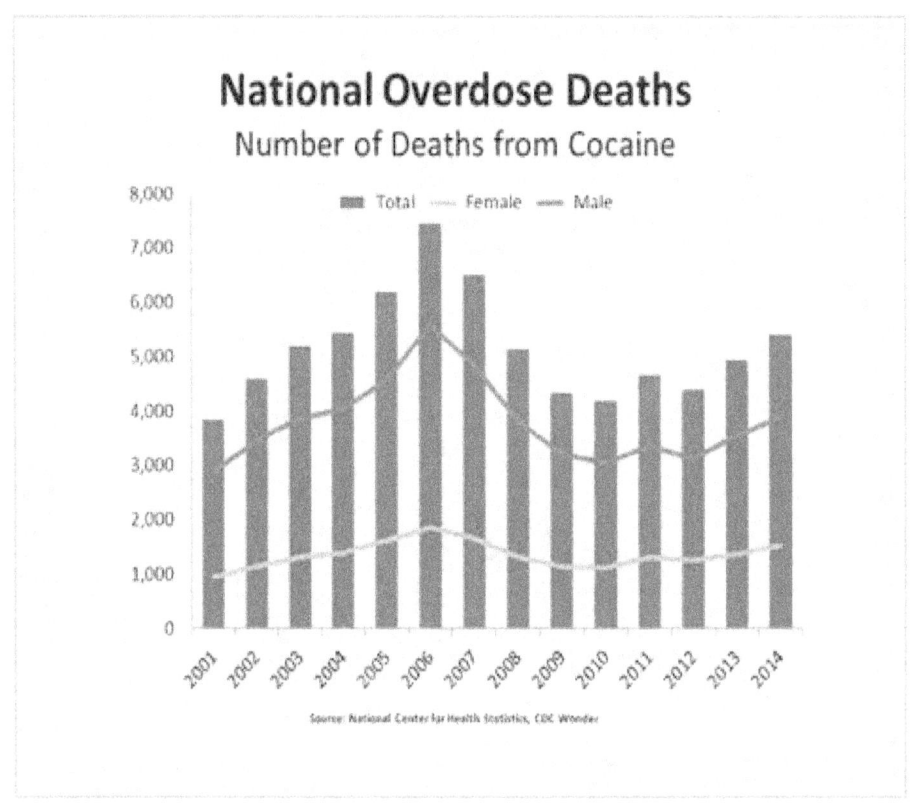

# How is cocaine used?

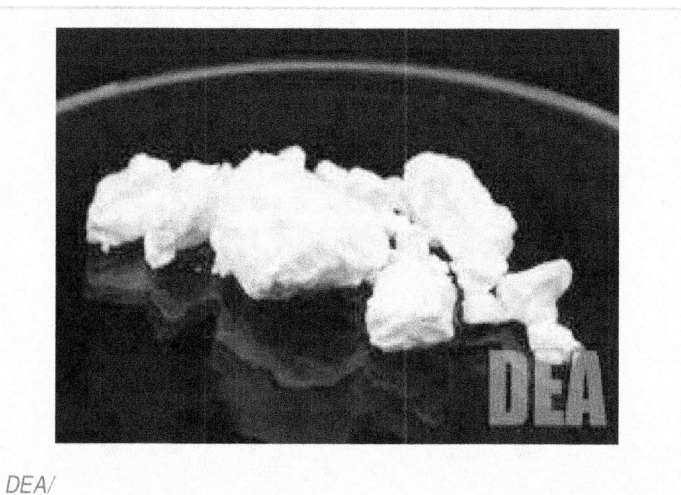

*Photo* by DEA/
Cocaine

Users primarily administer cocaine orally, intranasally, intravenously, or by inhalation. When people snort the drug (intranasal use), they inhale cocaine powder through the nostrils, where it is absorbed into the bloodstream through the nasal tissues. Users also may rub the drug onto their gums (oral use). Dissolving cocaine in water and injecting it (intravenous use) releases the drug directly into the bloodstream and heightens the intensity of its effects. When people smoke cocaine (inhalation), they inhale its vapor or smoke into the lungs, where absorption into the bloodstream is almost as rapid as by injection. This fast euphoric effect is one of the reasons that crack became enormously popular in the mid-1980s.[2]

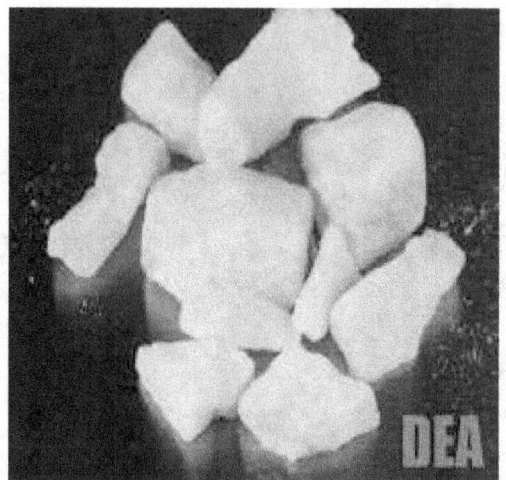

*Photo* by DEA/
Crack cocaine

Cocaine use ranges from occasional to repeated or compulsive use, with a variety of patterns between these extremes. Any route of administration can potentially lead to absorption of toxic amounts of cocaine, causing heart attacks, strokes, or seizures—all of which can result in sudden death.[2,7]

# How does cocaine produce its effects?

The brain's *mesolimbic dopamine system*, its reward pathway, is stimulated by all types of reinforcing stimuli, such as food, sex, and many drugs of abuse, including cocaine.[8] This pathway originates in a region of the midbrain called the ventral tegmental area and extends to the nucleus accumbens, one of the brain's key reward areas.[8] Besides reward, this circuit also regulates emotions and motivation.

In the normal communication process, dopamine is released by a neuron into the synapse (the small gap between two neurons), where it binds to specialized proteins called *dopamine receptors* on the neighboring neuron. By this process, dopamine acts as a chemical messenger, carrying a signal from neuron to neuron. Another specialized protein called a *transporter* removes dopamine from the synapse to be recycled for further use.[8]

Drugs of abuse can interfere with this normal communication process. For example, cocaine acts by binding to the dopamine transporter, blocking the removal of dopamine from the synapse. Dopamine then accumulates in the synapse to produce an amplified signal to the receiving neurons. This is what causes the euphoria commonly experienced immediately after taking the drug (see the video "Brain Reward: Understanding How the Brain Responds to Natural Rewards and Drugs of Abuse").

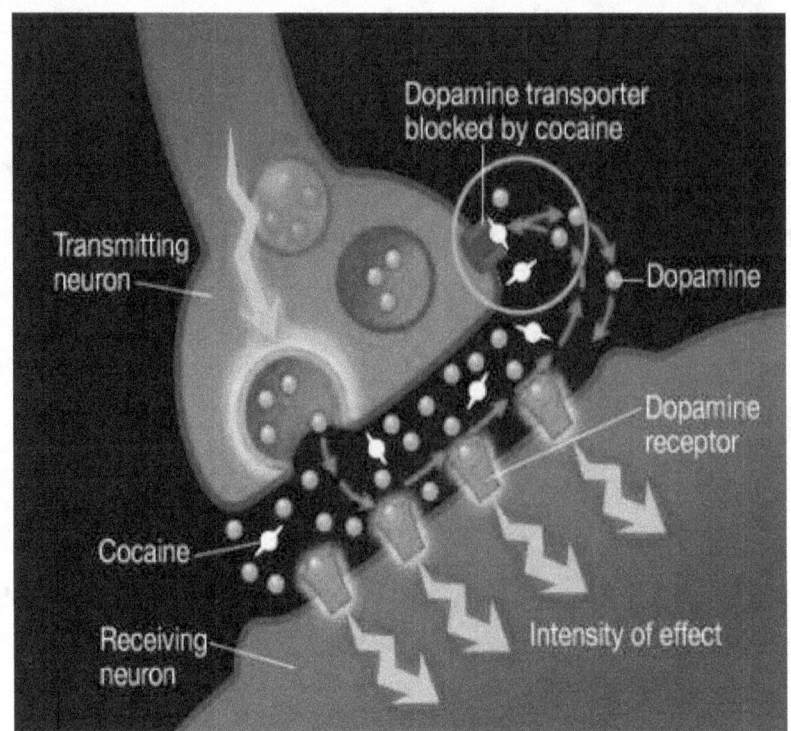

*Image by NIDA*

Cocaine in the brain: In the normal neural communication process, dopamine is released by a neuron into the synapse, where it can bind to dopamine receptors on neighboring neurons. Normally, dopamine is then recycled back into the transmitting neuron by a specialized protein called the dopamine transporter. If cocaine is present, it attaches to the dopamine transporter and blocks the normal recycling process, resulting in a buildup of dopamine in the synapse, which contributes to the pleasurable effects of cocaine.

# What are some ways that cocaine changes the brain?

Use of cocaine, like other drugs of abuse, induces long-term changes in the brain. Animal studies show that cocaine exposure can cause significant neuroadaptations in neurons that release the excitatory neurotransmitter glutamate.[9,10] Animals chronically exposed to cocaine demonstrate profound changes in glutamate neurotransmission—including how much is released and the level of receptor proteins—in the reward pathway, particularly the nucleus accumbens. The glutamate system may be an opportune target for anti-addiction medication development, with the goal of reversing the cocaine-induced neuroadaptations that contribute to the drive to use the drug.[9]

Although addiction researchers have focused on adaptations in the brain's reward system, drugs also affect the brain pathways that respond to stress. Stress can contribute to cocaine relapse, and cocaine use disorders frequently co-occur with stress-related disorders.[11] The stress circuits of the brain are distinct from the reward pathway, but research indicates that there are important ways that they overlap. The ventral tegmental area seems to act as a critical integration site in the brain that relays information about both stress and drug cues to other areas of the brain, including ones that drive cocaine seeking.[11] Animals that have received cocaine repeatedly are more likely to seek the drug in response to stress, and the more of the drug they have taken, the more stress affects this behavior.[11] Research suggests that cocaine elevates stress hormones, inducing neuroadaptations that further increase sensitivity to the drug and cues associated with it.[11]

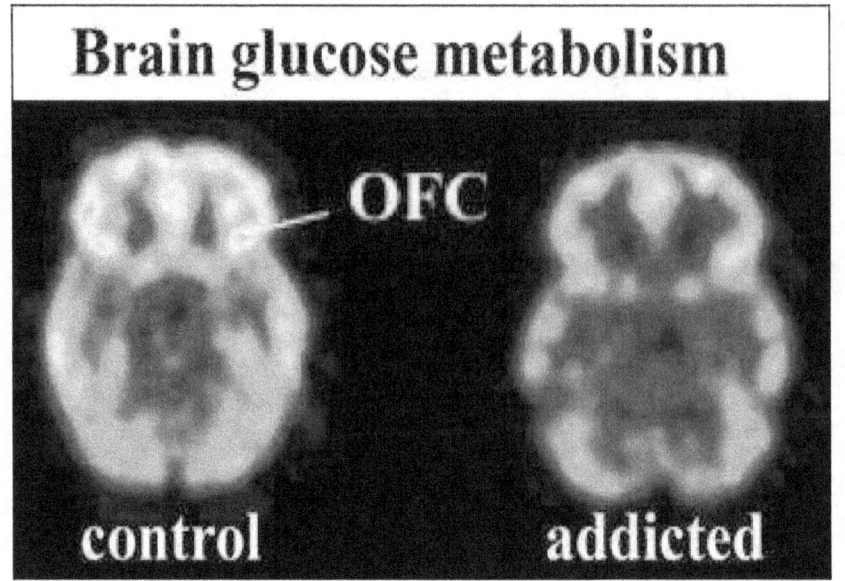

Brain images showing decreased glucose metabolism, which indicates reduced activity, in the orbitofrontal cortex (OFC) in a control subject (left) and a cocaine-addicted subject (right).
Volkow ND, Want G-J, Fowler JS, Tomasi D, Teland F. Addiction: beyond dopamine reward circuitry. *Proc Natl Acad Sci USA.* 2011;108(37):15037-15042.

Chronic cocaine exposure affects many other areas of the brain too. For example, animal research indicates that cocaine diminishes functioning in the orbitofrontal cortex (OFC), which appears to underlie the poor decision-making, inability to adapt to negative consequences of drug use, and lack of self-insight shown by people addicted to cocaine.[12] A study using optogenetic technology, which uses light to activate specific, genetically-modified neurons, found that stimulating the OFC restores adaptive learning in animals. This intriguing result suggests that strengthening OFC activity may be a good therapeutic approach to improve insight and awareness of the consequences of drug use among people addicted to cocaine.[13]

# What are the short-term effects of cocaine use?

Cocaine's effects appear almost immediately after a single dose and disappear within a few minutes to an hour. Small amounts of cocaine usually make the user feel euphoric, energetic, talkative, mentally alert, and hypersensitive to sight, sound, and touch. The drug can also temporarily decrease the need for food and sleep.[14] Some users find that cocaine helps them perform simple physical and intellectual tasks more quickly, although others experience the opposite effect.

The duration of cocaine's euphoric effects depend upon the route of administration. The faster the drug is absorbed, the more intense the resulting high, but also the shorter its duration. Snorting cocaine produces a relatively slow onset of the high, but it may last from 15 to 30 minutes. In contrast, the high from smoking is more immediate but may last only 5 to 10 minutes.[15]

Short-term physiological effects of cocaine use include constricted blood vessels; dilated pupils; and increased body temperature, heart rate, and blood pressure.[16] Large amounts of cocaine may intensify the user's high but can also lead to bizarre, erratic, and violent behavior. Some cocaine users report feelings of restlessness, irritability, anxiety, panic, and paranoia.[2] Users may also experience tremors, vertigo, and muscle twitches.[2]

Severe medical complications can occur with cocaine use. Some of the most frequent are cardiovascular effects, including disturbances in heart rhythm and heart attacks; neurological effects, including headaches, seizures, strokes, and coma; and gastrointestinal complications, including abdominal pain and nausea.[7] In rare instances, sudden death can occur on the first use of cocaine or unexpectedly thereafter. Cocaine-related deaths are often a result of cardiac arrest or seizures[2] (see "[National Overdose Deaths: Number of Deaths from Cocaine](#)"). Many cocaine users also use alcohol, and this combination can be particularly dangerous. The two substances react to produce cocaethylene, which may potentiate the toxic effects of cocaine and alcohol on the heart.[17] The combination of cocaine and heroin is also very dangerous. Users combine these drugs because the stimulating effects of cocaine are offset by the sedating effects of heroin; however, this can lead to taking a high dose of heroin without initially realizing it. Because cocaine's effects wear off sooner, this can lead to a heroin overdose, in which the user's respiration dangerously slows down or stops, possibly fatally.

# What are the long-term effects of cocaine use?

With repeated exposure to cocaine, the brain starts to adapt so that the reward pathway becomes less sensitive to natural reinforcers[10,18] (see "What Are Some Ways that Cocaine Changes the Brain?"). At the same time, circuits involved in stress become increasingly sensitive, leading to increased displeasure and negative moods when not taking the drug, which are signs of withdrawal. These combined effects make the user more likely to focus on seeking the drug instead of relationships, food, or other natural rewards.

With regular use, tolerance may develop so that higher doses, more frequent use of cocaine, or both are needed to produce the same level of pleasure and relief from withdrawal experienced initially.[10,18] At the same time, users can also develop sensitization, in which less cocaine is needed to produce anxiety, convulsions, or other toxic effects.[7] Tolerance to cocaine reward and sensitization to cocaine toxicity can increase the risk of overdose in a regular user.

Users take cocaine in binges, in which cocaine is used repeatedly and at increasingly higher doses. This can lead to increased irritability, restlessness, panic attacks, paranoia, and even a full-blown psychosis, in which the individual loses touch with reality and experiences auditory hallucinations.[2] With increasing doses or higher frequency of use, the risk of adverse psychological or physiological effects increases.[2,7] Animal research suggests that binging on cocaine during adolescence enhances sensitivity to the rewarding effects of cocaine and MDMA (Ecstasy or Molly).[19] Thus, binge use of cocaine during adolescence may further increase vulnerability to continued use of the drug among some people.

Specific routes of cocaine administration can produce their own adverse effects. Regularly snorting cocaine can lead to loss of sense of smell, nosebleeds, problems with swallowing, hoarseness, and an overall irritation of the nasal septum leading to a chronically inflamed, runny nose.[15] Smoking crack cocaine damages the lungs and can worsen asthma.[2,3] People who inject cocaine have puncture marks called tracks, most commonly in their forearms,[7] and they are at risk of contracting infectious diseases like HIV and hepatitis C (see "Why Are Cocaine Users at Risk for Contracting HIV and Hepatitis?"). They also may experience allergic reactions, either to the drug itself or to additives in street cocaine, which in severe cases can result in death.

Cocaine damages many other organs in the body. It reduces blood flow in the gastrointestinal tract, which can lead to tears and ulcerations.[7] Many chronic cocaine users lose their appetite and experience significant weight loss and malnourishment. Cocaine has significant and well-recognized toxic effects on the heart and cardiovascular system.[7,16,20] Chest pain that feels like a heart attack is common and sends many cocaine users to the emergency room.[7,20] Cocaine use is linked with increased risk of stroke,[16] as well as inflammation of the heart muscle, deterioration of the ability of the heart to contract, and aortic ruptures.[20]

In addition to the increased risk for stroke and seizures, other neurological problems can occur with long-term cocaine use.[7,18] There have been reports of *intracerebral hemorrhage*, or bleeding within the brain, and balloon-like bulges in the walls of cerebral blood vessels.[7,18] Movement disorders, including Parkinson's disease, may also occur after many years of cocaine use.[7] Generally, studies suggest that a wide range of cognitive functions are impaired with long-term cocaine use—such as sustaining attention, impulse inhibition, memory, making decisions involving rewards or punishments, and performing motor tasks.[14]

Former cocaine users are at high risk for relapse, even following long periods of abstinence. Research indicates that during periods of abstinence, the memory of the cocaine experience or exposure to cues associated with drug use can trigger strong cravings, which can lead to relapse.[21]

# Why are cocaine users at risk for contracting HIV/AIDS and hepatitis?

Drug intoxication and addiction can compromise judgment and decision-making and potentially lead to risky sexual behavior, including trading sex for drugs, and needle sharing. This increases a cocaine user's risk for contracting infectious diseases such as HIV and hepatitis C (HCV).[22] There are no vaccines to prevent HIV or HCV infections.

Studies that examine patterns of HIV infection and progression have demonstrated that cocaine use accelerates HIV infection.[23] Research indicates that cocaine impairs immune cell function,[24] promotes replication of the HIV virus, and potentiates the damaging effects of HIV on different types of cells in the brain and spinal cord, resulting in further damage.[23] Studies also suggest that cocaine use accelerates the development of NeuroAIDS, neurological conditions associated with HIV infection. Symptoms of NeuroAIDS include memory loss, movement problems, and vision impairment.[23]

Cocaine users with HIV often have advanced progression of the disease, with increased viral load and accelerated decreases in CD4+ cell counts. Infection with HIV increases risk for co-infection with HCV, a virus that affects the liver.[24] Co-infection can lead to serious illnesses—including problems with the immune system and neurologic conditions. Liver complications are very common, with many co-infected individuals dying of chronic liver disease and cancer.[22] Although the link between injection drug use and HIV/HCV is well established, more studies are needed to understand the molecular mechanisms underlying this increased risk of co-infection in non-injecting substance users.[24]

The interaction of substance use, HIV, and hepatitis may accelerate disease progression. For example, HIV speeds the course of HCV infection by accelerating the progression of hepatitis-associated liver disease.[24] Research has linked HIV/HCV co-infection with increased mortality when compared to either infection alone.[24] Substance use and co-infection likely negatively influence HIV disease progression and the ability of the body to marshal an immune response.[24]

Patients with HIV/HCV co-infection can benefit from substance abuse treatment and antiretroviral therapies, when closely monitored.[22] Antiretroviral treatment is not effective for everyone and can have significant side effects, necessitating close medical supervision. Testing for HIV and HCV is recommended for any individual who has ever injected drugs, since the disease is highly transmissible via injection.

# What are the effects of maternal cocaine use?

Most women who are addicted to cocaine are of childbearing age. Estimates suggest that about 5 percent of pregnant women use one or more addictive substances,[25] and there are around 750,000 cocaine-exposed pregnancies every year.[26] Although women may be reluctant to report substance use patterns because of social stigma and fear of losing custody of their children, they should be aware that drug use while pregnant is associated with specific risks that may be reduced with appropriate care.

Cocaine use during pregnancy is associated with maternal migraines and seizures, premature membrane rupture, and separation of the placental lining from the uterus prior to delivery.[25] Pregnancy is accompanied by normal cardiovascular changes, and cocaine use exacerbates these—sometimes leading to serious problems with high blood pressure (hypertensive crises), spontaneous miscarriage, preterm labor, and difficult delivery.[26] Cocaine-using pregnant women must receive appropriate medical and psychological care—including addiction treatment—to reduce these risks.[25]

Sex-specific addiction treatment and comprehensive services—including prenatal care, mental health counseling, vocational/employment assistance, and parenting skills training—can promote drug abstinence and other positive health behaviors.[27] Motivational incentives/contingency management (see "[Behavioral Interventions]") as an adjunct to other addiction treatment is a particularly promising strategy to engage women in prenatal care and counseling for substance use.[28]

It is difficult to estimate the full extent of the consequences of maternal drug use and to determine the specific hazard of a particular drug to the unborn child. This is because multiple factors—such as the amount and number of *all* drugs used, including nicotine or alcohol; extent of prenatal care; exposure to violence in the environment; socioeconomic conditions; maternal nutrition; other health conditions; and exposure to sexually transmitted diseases—can all interact to influence maternal and child outcomes.[26,29,30] Similarly, parenting styles, quality of care during early childhood, exposure to violence, and continued parental drug use are strong environmental factors influencing outcomes.[31,32]

Babies born to mothers who use cocaine during pregnancy are often prematurely delivered, have low birth weights and smaller head circumferences, and are shorter in length than babies born to mothers who do not use cocaine.[26,29,30] Dire predictions of reduced intelligence and social skills in babies born to mothers who used crack cocaine while pregnant during the 1980s—so-called "crack babies"—were grossly exaggerated. However, the fact that most of these children do not show serious overt deficits should not be overinterpreted to indicate that there is no cause for concern.

Using sophisticated technologies, scientists are now finding that exposure to cocaine during fetal development may lead to subtle, yet significant, later deficits in some children.[31,32] These include behavior problems (e.g., difficulties with self-regulation) and deficits in some aspects of cognitive performance, information processing, and sustained attention to tasks—abilities that are important for the realization of a child's full potential.[32,33] Some deficits persist into the later years, with prenatally exposed adolescents showing increased risk for subtle problems with language and memory.[34] Brain scans in teens suggests that at-rest functioning of some brain regions—including areas involved in attention, planning, and language—may differ from that of non-exposed peers.[35] More research is needed on the long-term effects of prenatal cocaine exposure.

# How is cocaine addiction treated?

In 2013, cocaine accounted for almost 6 percent of all admissions to drug abuse treatment programs. The majority of individuals (68 percent in 2013) who seek treatment for cocaine use smoke crack and are likely to be polydrug users, meaning they use more than one substance.[36] Those who provide treatment for cocaine use should recognize that drug addiction is a complex disease involving changes in the brain as well as a wide range of social, familial, and other environmental factors; therefore, treatment of cocaine addiction must address this broad context as well as any other co-occurring mental disorders that require additional behavioral or pharmacological interventions.

## Pharmacological Approaches

Presently, there are no medications approved by the U.S. Food and Drug Administration to treat cocaine addiction, though researchers are exploring a variety of neurobiological targets. Past research has primarily focused on dopamine, but scientists have also found that cocaine use induces changes in the brain related to other neurotransmitters—including serotonin, gamma-aminobutyric acid (GABA), norepinephrine, and glutamate.[37] Researchers are currently testing medications that act at the dopamine $D_3$ receptor, a subtype of dopamine receptor that is abundant in the emotion and reward centers of the brain.[38] Other research is testing compounds (e.g., *N*-acetylcysteine) that restore the balance between excitatory (glutamate) and inhibitory (GABA) neurotransmission, which is disrupted by long-term cocaine use.[39] Research in animals is also looking at medications (e.g., lorcaserin) that act at serotonin receptors.[40]

Several medications marketed for other diseases show promise in reducing cocaine use within controlled clinical trials. Among these, disulfiram, which is used to treat alcoholism, has shown the most promise. Scientists do not yet know exactly how disulfiram reduces cocaine use, though its effects may be related to its ability to inhibit an enzyme that converts dopamine to norepinephrine. However, disulfiram does not work for everyone. Pharmacogenetic studies are revealing variants in the gene that encodes the DBH enzyme and seems to influence disulfiram's effectiveness in reducing cocaine use.[41–43] Knowing a patient's *DBH* genotype could help predict whether disulfiram would be an effective pharmacotherapy for cocaine dependence in that person.[41–43]

Finally, researchers have developed and conducted early tests on a cocaine vaccine that could help reduce the risk of relapse. The vaccine stimulates the immune system to create cocaine-specific antibodies that bind to cocaine, preventing it from getting into the brain.[44] In addition to showing the vaccine's safety, a clinical trial found that patients who attained high antibody levels significantly reduced cocaine use.[45] However, only 38 percent of the vaccinated subjects attained sufficient antibody levels and for only 2 months.[45]

Researchers are working to improve the cocaine vaccine by enhancing the strength of binding to cocaine and its ability to elicit antibodies.[44,46] New vaccine technologies, including gene transfer to boost the specificity and level of antibodies produced or enhance the metabolism of cocaine, may also improve the effectiveness of this treatment.[47] A pharmacogenetics study with a small number of patients suggests that individuals with a particular genotype respond well to the cocaine vaccine—an intriguing finding that requires more research.[48]

In addition to treatments for addiction, researchers are developing medical interventions to address the acute emergencies that result from cocaine overdose. One approach being explored is the use of genetically engineered human enzymes involved in the breakdown of cocaine, which would counter the behavioral and toxic effects of a cocaine overdose.[49] Currently, researchers are testing and refining these enzymes in animal research, with the ultimate goal of moving to clinical trials.[49]

## Behavioral Interventions

Many behavioral treatments for cocaine addiction have proven to be effective in both residential and outpatient settings. Indeed, behavioral therapies are often the only available and effective treatments for many drug problems, including stimulant addictions. However, the integration of behavioral and pharmacological treatments may ultimately prove to be the most effective approach.[50]

One form of behavioral therapy that is showing positive results in people with cocaine use disorders is contingency management (CM), also called motivational incentives. Programs use a voucher or prize-based system that rewards patients who abstain from cocaine and other drugs. On the basis of drug-free urine tests, the patients earn points, or chips, which can be exchanged for items that encourage healthy living, such as a gym membership, movie tickets, or dinner at a local restaurant. CM may be particularly useful for helping patients achieve initial abstinence from cocaine and stay in treatment.[39,50–52] This approach has recently been shown to be practical and effective in community treatment programs.[51]

Research indicates that CM benefits diverse populations of cocaine users. For example, studies show that cocaine-dependent pregnant women and women with young children who participated in a CM program as an adjunct to other substance use disorder treatment were able to stay abstinent longer than those who received an equivalent amount of vouchers with no behavioral requirements.[28] Patients participating in CM treatment for cocaine use who also experienced psychiatric symptoms—such as depression, emotional distress, and hostility—showed a significant reduction in these problems, probably related to reductions in cocaine use.[53]

Cognitive-behavioral therapy (CBT) is an effective approach for preventing relapse. This approach helps patients develop critical skills that support long-term abstinence—including the ability to recognize the situations in which they are most likely to use cocaine, avoid these situations, and cope more effectively with a range of problems associated with drug use. This therapy can also be used in conjunction with other treatments, thereby maximizing the benefits of both.[50]

Recently, researchers developed a computerized form of CBT (CBT4CBT) that patients use in a private room of a clinic.[54–56] This interactive multimedia program closely follows the key lessons and skill-development activities of in-person CBT in a series of modules. Movies present examples and information that support the development of coping skills; quizzes, games, and homework assignments reinforce the lessons and provide opportunities to practice skills.[54–56] Studies have shown that adding CBT4CBT to weekly counseling boosted abstinence[54] and increased treatment success rates up to 6 months after treatment.[55]

Therapeutic communities (TCs)—drug-free residences in which people in recovery from substance use disorders help each other to understand and change their behaviors—can be an effective treatment for people who use drugs, including cocaine.[57] TCs may require a 6- to 12-month stay and can include onsite vocational rehabilitation and other supportive services that focus on successful re-integration of the individual into society. TCs can also provide support in other important areas—improving legal, employment, and mental health outcomes.[57,58]

Regardless of the specific type of substance use disorder treatment, it is important that patients receive services that match all of their treatment needs. For example, an unemployed patient would benefit from vocational rehabilitation or career counseling along with addiction treatment. Patients with marital problems may need couples counseling. Once inpatient treatment ends, ongoing support—also called aftercare—can help people avoid relapse. Research indicates that people who are committed to abstinence, engage in self-help behaviors, and believe that they have the ability to refrain from using cocaine (self-efficacy) are more likely to abstain.[59] Aftercare serves to reinforce these traits and address problems that may increase vulnerability to relapse, including depression and declining self-efficacy.[59]

Scientists have found promising results from telephone-based counseling as a low-cost method to deliver aftercare. For example, people who misused stimulants who participated in seven sessions of telephone counseling showed decreasing drug use during the first 3 months, whereas those who did not receive calls increased their use.[60] Voucher incentives can boost patients' willingness to participate in telephone aftercare, doubling the number of sessions received according to one study.[61]

Community-based recovery groups—such as Cocaine Anonymous—that use a

12-step program can also be helpful in maintaining abstinence. Participants may benefit from the supportive fellowship and from sharing with those experiencing common problems and issues.[62]

# How is cutting-edge science helping us better understand addiction?

Two cutting-edge areas of science, genetics and brain imaging, are significantly advancing our understanding of cocaine addiction.

Researchers estimate that genetics contributes 42 to 79 percent of the risk for cocaine use and dependence.[63] Of course, with a complex disease such as addiction, many different genes are involved, and their expression can be influenced by the environment. There appears to be significant overlap in the genes that put people at risk for all addictive substances, perhaps indicating a common biological pathway for addiction regardless of the drug.[63]

In genome-wide association studies (GWAS), researchers examine whether certain gene variants are more frequently found in people with a substance use disorder, which eventually might help identify those at increased risk for drug addiction.[64,65] Identifying genes linked to addiction is only the first step. Candidate-gene research examines the links between substance use and specific genes that encode proteins that appear to be related to addiction. For example, researchers have found connections between various aspects of cocaine addiction and the genes that encode for particular dopamine receptors and the enzymes that break down this neurotransmitter.[63]

Because environmental factors typically shape the impact of genes on disease risk, researchers must also identify how particular gene-by-environment interactions influence the course of addiction.[63] Research in the field of *epigenetics* is uncovering how the environment induces long-term changes in gene expression—influencing the pattern of gene expression—without altering the DNA sequence.[66]

In animal research, scientists are determining how long-term cocaine exposure changes gene expression in the brain, particularly in the reward pathway. Studies have linked specific cocaine-induced epigenetic changes to neuroadaptations[67] and behavioral hallmarks of addiction, such as sensitivity to cocaine's rewarding effects.[66,67] The epigenetic changes induced by cocaine can be passed to the next generation, even if the drug exposure does not occur prenatally.[68] Although much more genetic and epigenetic research is needed, understanding addiction at the molecular level offers great promise for improving diagnosis, for example by discovering biomarkers for disease severity or treatment response.[66]

Although more research is needed, brain-imaging might be used to detect biomarkers for drug addiction vulnerability, as these technologies have yielded insights into the processes underlying craving and how medications may quell the brain's response to cocaine cues.[69] A relatively new neuroimaging technology called default-mode or resting-state functional magnetic resonance imaging (rs-fMRI) reveals brain activity when people are alert but not performing a particular task; researchers use this technique to compare functional brain networks of people who have used cocaine for a long time and those who have not. These studies suggest that there is reduced connectivity between various brain circuits[70–72] and between the two hemispheres[73] among people with cocaine dependence. Researchers have also correlated reduced connectivity between particular brain circuits with important addiction-related behaviors, including risk for relapse[71] and impulsivity.[72]

Neuroimaging technologies are also documenting how the brains of cocaine users may recover after periods of abstinence. For example, these techniques indicate that years of cocaine use are associated with reduced grey matter in particular brain regions. However, people who maintained cocaine abstinence for approximately 9 months showed grey matter levels similar to or greater than those of people who had never used the drug.[74] Further analysis indicated that the increased grey matter occurred in regions other than the ones altered by cocaine use, suggesting that the neurobiological changes involved in recovery are more complex than simply reversing the changes related to addiction.[74] The researchers also found that increased grey matter volume in brain regions involved with behavioral control were associated with longer duration of abstinence.[74]

fMRI technologies have also revealed that abstinence from cocaine has important, restorative effects on the brain. Although current cocaine users demonstrated reduced brain activity in a brain circuit that mediates response inhibition during a motor control task, individuals who had attained abstinence for an average of 8 months showed similar patterns of activation and levels of performance to those who had never used the drug.[75] The results suggest that abstinence helps restore the functioning of this brain circuit.

Researchers are engaged in several large-scale, collaborative projects to map the human connectome, which is the brain's network of interconnected circuits. For example, the National Institutes of Health supports the Human Connectome Project to generate maps of the developing, adult, and aging brain. By having a map of the typical brain, scientists will further understand how neural functioning differs in behavioral disorders—knowledge that will drive improved diagnostics and treatments.

# References

1. Calatayud J, González A. History of the development and evolution of local anesthesia since the coca leaf. *Anesthesiology*. 2003;98(6):1503-1508.

2. Goldstein RA, DesLauriers C, Burda AM. Cocaine: history, social implications, and toxicity–a review. *Dis–Mon DM*. 2009;55(1):6-38. doi:10.1016/j.disamonth.2008.10.002.

3. Drent M, Wijnen P, Bast A. Interstitial lung damage due to cocaine abuse: pathogenesis, pharmacogenomics and therapy. *Curr Med Chem*. 2012;19(33):5607-5611.

4. Center for Behavioral Health Statistics and Quality (CBHSQ). *Behavioral Health Trends in the United States: Results from the 2014 National Survey on Drug Use and Health*. Rockville, MD: Substance Abuse and Mental Health Services Administration; 2015. HHS Publication No. SMA 15-4927, NSDUH Series H-50.

5. Johnston L, O'Malley P, Miech R, Bachman J, Schulenberg J. *Monitoring the Future National Survey Results on Drug Use: 1975-2015: Overview: Key Findings on Adolescent Drug Use*. Ann Arbor, MI: Institute for Social Research, The University of Michigan; 2015.

6. Center for Behavioral Health Statistics and Quality (CBHSQ). *Drug Abuse Warning Network: 2011: Selected Tables of National Estimates of Drug-Related Emergency Department Visits*. Rockville, MD: Substance Abuse and Mental Health Services Administration; 2013.

7. Riezzo I, Fiore C, De Carlo D, et al. Side effects of cocaine abuse: multiorgan toxicity and pathological consequences. *Curr Med Chem*. 2012;19(33):5624-5646.

8. Baik J-H. Dopamine signaling in reward-related behaviors. *Front Neural Circuits*. 2013;7. doi:10.3389/fncir.2013.00152.

9. Schmidt HD, Pierce RC. Cocaine-induced neuroadaptations in glutamate transmission: potential therapeutic targets for craving and addiction. *Ann N Y Acad Sci*. 2010;1187:35-75. doi:10.1111/j.1749-6632.2009.05144.x.

10. Wolf ME. The Bermuda Triangle of cocaine-induced neuroadaptations.

*Trends Neurosci.* 2010;33(9):391-398. doi:10.1016/j.tins.2010.06.003.

11. Mantsch JR, Vranjkovic O, Twining RC, Gasser PJ, McReynolds JR, Blacktop JM. Neurobiological mechanisms that contribute to stress-related cocaine use. *Neuropharmacology.* 2014;76, Part B:383-394. doi:10.1016/j.neuropharm.2013.07.021.

12. Lucantonio F, Stalnaker TA, Shaham Y, Niv Y, Schoenbaum G. The impact of orbitofrontal dysfunction on cocaine addiction. *Nat Neurosci.* 2012;15(3):358-366. doi:10.1038/nn.3014.

13. Lucantonio F, Takahashi YK, Hoffman AF, et al. Orbitofrontal activation restores insight lost after cocaine use. *Nat Neurosci.* 2014;17(8):1092-1099. doi:10.1038/nn.3763.

14. Spronk DB, van Wel JHP, Ramaekers JG, Verkes RJ. Characterizing the cognitive effects of cocaine: a comprehensive review. *Neurosci Biobehav Rev.* 2013;37(8):1838-1859. doi:10.1016/j.neubiorev.2013.07.003.

15. Advokat C, Comaty J, Julien R. *Julien's Primer of Drug Action.* 13th ed. New York, NY: Worth Publishers; 2014.

16. Fonseca AC, Ferro JM. Drug abuse and stroke. *Curr Neurol Neurosci Rep.* 2013;13(2):325. doi:10.1007/s11910-012-0325-0.

17. Pennings EJM, Leccese AP, Wolff FA de. Effects of concurrent use of alcohol and cocaine. *Addict Abingdon Engl.* 2002;97(7):773-783.

18. Büttner A. Neuropathological alterations in cocaine abuse. *Curr Med Chem.* 2012;19(33):5597-5600.

19. Mateos-García A, Roger-Sánchez C, Rodriguez-Arias M, et al. Higher sensitivity to the conditioned rewarding effects of cocaine and MDMA in High-Novelty-Seekers mice exposed to a cocaine binge during adolescence. *Psychopharmacology (Berl).* 2015;232(1):101-113. doi:10.1007/s00213-014-3642-y.

20. Maraj S, Figueredo VM, Lynn Morris D. Cocaine and the heart. *Clin Cardiol.* 2010;33(5):264-269. doi:10.1002/clc.20746.

21. Sinha R. The clinical neurobiology of drug craving. *Curr Opin Neurobiol.* 2013;23(4):649-654. doi:10.1016/j.conb.2013.05.001.

22. Khalsa JH, Elkashef A. Interventions for HIV and hepatitis C virus infections in recreational drug users. *Clin Infect Dis.* 2010;50(11):1505-1511. doi:10.1086/652447.

23. Buch S, Yao H, Guo M, et al. Cocaine and HIV-1 interplay in CNS: cellular and molecular mechanisms. *Curr HIV Res.* 2012;10(5):425-428.

24. Parikh N, Nonnemacher MR, Pirrone V, Block T, Mehta A, Wigdahl B. Substance abuse, HIV-1 and hepatitis. *Curr HIV Res.* 2012;10(7):557-571.

25. Wendell AD. Overview and epidemiology of substance abuse in pregnancy. *Clin Obstet Gynecol.* 2013;56(1):91-96. doi:10.1097/GRF.0b013e31827feeb9.

26. Cain MA, Bornick P, Whiteman V. The maternal, fetal, and neonatal effects of cocaine exposure in pregnancy. *Clin Obstet Gynecol.* 2013;56(1):124-132. doi:10.1097/GRF.0b013e31827ae167.

27. Hull L, May J, Farrell-Moore D, Svikis DS. Treatment of cocaine abuse during pregnancy: translating research to clinical practice. *Curr Psychiatry Rep.* 2010;12(5):454-461. doi:10.1007/s11920-010-0138-2.

28. Schottenfeld RS, Moore B, Pantalon MV. Contingency management with community reinforcement approach or twelve-step facilitation drug counseling for cocaine dependent pregnant women or women with young children. *Drug Alcohol Depend.* 2011;118(1):48-55. doi:10.1016/j.drugalcdep.2011.02.019.

29. Behnke M, Smith VC, Abuse C on S, Newborn C on FA. Prenatal substance abuse: short- and long-term effects on the exposed fetus. *Pediatrics.* 2013;131(3):e1009-e1024. doi:10.1542/peds.2012-3931.

30. Gouin K, Murphy K, Shah PS, Knowledge Synthesis group on Determinants of Low Birth Weight and Preterm Births. Effects of cocaine use during pregnancy on low birthweight and preterm birth: systematic review and metaanalyses. *Am J Obstet Gynecol.* 2011;204(4):340.e1-e12. doi:10.1016/j.ajog.2010.11.013.

31. Lambert BL, Bauer CR. Developmental and behavioral consequences of prenatal cocaine exposure: a review. *J Perinatol Off J Calif Perinat Assoc.* 2012;32(11):819-828. doi:10.1038/jp.2012.90.

32. Lester BM, Lagasse LL. Children of addicted women. *J Addict Dis*. 2010;29(2):259-276. doi:10.1080/10550881003684921.

33. Ackerman JP, Riggins T, Black MM. A review of the effects of prenatal cocaine exposure among school-aged children. *Pediatrics*. 2010;125(3):554-565. doi:10.1542/peds.2009-0637.

34. Buckingham-Howes S, Berger SS, Scaletti LA, Black MM. Systematic review of prenatal cocaine exposure and adolescent development. *Pediatrics*. 2013;131(6):e1917-e1936. doi:10.1542/peds.2012-0945.

35. Li K, Zhu D, Guo L, et al. Connectomics signatures of prenatal cocaine exposure affected adolescent brains. *Hum Brain Mapp*. 2013;34(10):2494-2510. doi:10.1002/hbm.22082.

36. Center for Behavioral Health Statistics and Quality (CBHSQ). *Treatment Episode Data Set (TEDS): 2003-2013. National Admissions to Substance Abuse Treatment Services.* Rockville, MD: Substance Abuse and Mental Health Services Administration; 2015. BHSIS Series S-75, HHS Publication No. (SMA) 15-4934.

37. Shorter D, Domingo CB, Kosten TR. Emerging drugs for the treatment of cocaine use disorder: a review of neurobiological targets and pharmacotherapy. *Expert Opin Emerg Drugs*. 2015;20(1):15-29. doi:10.1517/14728214.2015.985203.

38. Karila L, Reynaud M, Aubin H-J, et al. Pharmacological treatments for cocaine dependence: is there something new? *Curr Pharm Des*. 2011;17(14):1359-1368.

39. Kampman KM. What's new in the treatment of cocaine addiction? *Curr Psychiatry Rep*. 2010;12(5):441-447. doi:10.1007/s11920-010-0143-5.

40. Harvey-Lewis C, Li Z, Higgins GA, Fletcher PJ. The 5-HT2C receptor agonist lorcaserin reduces cocaine self-administration, reinstatement of cocaine-seeking and cocaine induced locomotor activity. *Neuropharmacology*. 2016;101:237-245. doi:10.1016/j.neuropharm.2015.09.028.

41. Shorter D, Nielsen DA, Huang W, Harding MJ, Hamon SC, Kosten TR. Pharmacogenetic randomized trial for cocaine abuse: disulfiram and 1A-adrenoceptor gene variation. *Eur Neuropsychopharmacol J Eur Coll Neuropsychopharmacol*. 2013;23(11):1401-1407.

doi:10.1016/j.euroneuro.2013.05.014.

42. Spellicy CJ, Kosten TR, Hamon SC, Harding MJ, Nielsen DA. ANKK1 and DRD2 pharmacogenetics of disulfiram treatment for cocaine abuse. *Pharmacogenet Genomics*. 2013;23(7):333-340. doi:10.1097/FPC.0b013e328361c39d.

43. Kosten TR, Wu G, Huang W, et al. Pharmacogenetic randomized trial for cocaine abuse: disulfiram and dopamine -hydroxylase. *Biol Psychiatry*. 2013;73(3):219-224. doi:10.1016/j.biopsych.2012.07.011.

44. Kosten TR, Domingo CB. Can you vaccinate against substance abuse? *Expert Opin Biol Ther*. 2013;13(8):1093-1097. doi:10.1517/14712598.2013.791278.

45. Martell BA, Orson FM, Poling J, et al. Cocaine vaccine for the treatment of cocaine dependence in methadone-maintained patients: a randomized, double-blind, placebo-controlled efficacy trial. *Arch Gen Psychiatry*. 2009;66(10):1116-1123. doi:10.1001/archgenpsychiatry.2009.128.

46. Cai X, Tsuchikama K, Janda KD. Modulating cocaine vaccine potency through hapten fluorination. *J Am Chem Soc*. 2013;135(8):2971-2974. doi:10.1021/ja400356g.

47. Brimijoin S, Shen X, Orson F, Kosten T. Prospects, promise and problems on the road to effective vaccines and related therapies for substance abuse. *Expert Rev Vaccines*. 2013;12(3):323-332. doi:10.1586/erv.13.1.

48. Nielsen DA, Hamon SC, Kosten TR. The -opioid receptor gene as a predictor of response in a cocaine vaccine clinical trial. *Psychiatr Genet*. 2013;23(6):225-232. doi:10.1097/YPG.0000000000000008.

49. Schindler CW, Goldberg SR. Accelerating cocaine metabolism as an approach to the treatment of cocaine abuse and toxicity. *Future Med Chem*. 2012;4(2):163-175. doi:10.4155/fmc.11.181.

50. Penberthy JK, Ait-Daoud N, Vaughan M, Fanning T. Review of treatment for cocaine dependence. *Curr Drug Abuse Rev*. 2010;3(1):49-62.

51. Petry NM, Barry D, Alessi SM, Rounsaville BJ, Carroll KM. A randomized trial adapting contingency management targets based on initial abstinence status of cocaine-dependent patients. *J Consult Clin Psychol*.

2012;80(2):276-285. doi:10.1037/a0026883.

52. Schierenberg A, van Amsterdam J, van den Brink W, Goudriaan AE. Efficacy of contingency management for cocaine dependence treatment: a review of the evidence. *Curr Drug Abuse Rev*. 2012;5(4):320-331.

53. Petry NM, Alessi SM, Rash CJ. Contingency management treatments decrease psychiatric symptoms. *J Consult Clin Psychol*. 2013;81(5):926-931. doi:10.1037/a0032499.

54. Carroll KM, Ball SA, Martino S, et al. Computer-assisted delivery of cognitive-behavioral therapy for addiction: a randomized trial of CBT4CBT. *Am J Psychiatry*. 2008;165(7):881-888. doi:10.1176/appi.ajp.2008.07111835.

55. Carroll KM, Ball SA, Martino S, Nich C, Babuscio TA, Rounsaville BJ. Enduring effects of a computer-assisted training program for cognitive behavioral therapy: a 6-month follow-up of CBT4CBT. *Drug Alcohol Depend*. 2009;100(1-2):178-181. doi:10.1016/j.drugalcdep.2008.09.015.

56. Carroll KM, Kiluk BD, Nich C, et al. Computer-assisted delivery of cognitive-behavioral therapy: efficacy and durability of CBT4CBT among cocaine-dependent individuals maintained on methadone. *Am J Psychiatry*. 2014;171(4):436-444. doi:10.1176/appi.ajp.2013.13070987.

57. Vanderplasschen W, Colpaert K, Autrique M, et al. Therapeutic communities for addictions: a review of their effectiveness from a recovery-oriented perspective. *Sci World J*. 2013;2013, 2013:e427817. doi:10.1155/2013/427817.

58. Leon GD. Is the therapeutic community an evidence based treatment? What the evidence says. *Ther Communities Int Jdournal Ther Support Organ*. 2010;31(2):104-128.

59. McKay JR, Van Horn D, Rennert L, Drapkin M, Ivey M, Koppenhaver J. Factors in sustained recovery from cocaine dependence. *J Subst Abuse Treat*. 2013;45(2):163-172. doi:10.1016/j.jsat.2013.02.007.

60. Farabee D, Cousins SJ, Brecht M-L, et al. A comparison of four telephone-based counseling styles for recovering stimulant users. *Psychol Addict Behav*. 2013;27(1):223-229. doi:10.1037/a0029572.

61. Van Horn DHA, Drapkin M, Ivey M, et al. Voucher incentives increase treatment participation in telephone-based continuing care for cocaine dependence. *Drug Alcohol Depend*. 2011;114(2-3):225-228. doi:10.1016/j.drugalcdep.2010.09.007.

62. Donovan DM, Daley DC, Brigham GS, et al. Stimulant abuser groups to engage in 12-step: a multisite trial in the National Institute on Drug Abuse Clinical Trials Network. *J Subst Abuse Treat*. 2013;44(1):103-114. doi:10.1016/j.jsat.2012.04.004.

63. Agrawal A, Verweij KJH, Gillespie NA, et al. The genetics of addiction-a translational perspective. *Transl Psychiatry*. 2012;2:e140. doi:10.1038/tp.2012.54.

64. Drgon T, Zhang P-W, Johnson C, et al. Genome wide association for addiction: replicated results and comparisons of two analytic approaches. *PloS One*. 2010;5(1):e8832. doi:10.1371/journal.pone.0008832.

65. Kreek MJ, Levran O, Reed B, Schlussman SD, Zhou Y, Butelman ER. Opiate addiction and cocaine addiction: underlying molecular neurobiology and genetics. *J Clin Invest*. 2012;122(10):3387-3393. doi:10.1172/JCI60390.

66. Nestler EJ. Epigenetic mechanisms of drug addiction. *Neuropharmacology*. 2014;76 Pt B:259-268. doi:10.1016/j.neuropharm.2013.04.004.

67. Schmidt HD, McGinty JF, West AE, Sadri-Vakili G. Epigenetics and psychostimulant addiction. *Cold Spring Harb Perspect Med*. 2013;3(3):a012047. doi:10.1101/cshperspect.a012047.

68. Vassoler FM, Sadri-Vakili G. Mechanisms of transgenerational inheritance of addictive-like behaviors. *Neuroscience*. 2014;264:198-206. doi:10.1016/j.neuroscience.2013.07.064.

69. Young KA, Franklin TR, Roberts DCS, et al. Nipping cue reactivity in the bud: baclofen prevents limbic activation elicited by subliminal drug cues. *J Neurosci Off J Soc Neurosci*. 2014;34(14):5038-5043. doi:10.1523/JNEUROSCI.4977-13.2014.

70. Gu H, Salmeron BJ, Ross TJ, et al. Mesocorticolimbic circuits are impaired in chronic cocaine users as demonstrated by resting-state functional connectivity. *NeuroImage*. 2010;53(2):593-601. doi:10.1016/j.neuroimage.2010.06.066.

71. McHugh MJ, Demers CH, Salmeron BJ, Devous MD, Stein EA, Adinoff B. Cortico-amygdala coupling as a marker of early relapse risk in cocaine-addicted individuals. *Front Psychiatry*. 2014;5:16. doi:10.3389/fpsyt.2014.00016.

72. Wisner KM, Patzelt EH, Lim KO, MacDonald AW. An intrinsic connectivity network approach to insula-derived dysfunctions among cocaine users. *Am J Drug Alcohol Abuse*. 2013;39(6):403-413. doi:10.3109/00952990.2013.848211.

73. Kelly C, Zuo X-N, Gotimer K, et al. Reduced interhemispheric resting state functional connectivity in cocaine addiction. *Biol Psychiatry*. 2011;69(7):684-692. doi:10.1016/j.biopsych.2010.11.022.

74. Connolly CG, Bell RP, Foxe JJ, Garavan H. Dissociated grey matter changes with prolonged addiction and extended abstinence in cocaine users. *PLoS ONE*. 2013;8(3):e59645. doi:10.1371/journal.pone.0059645.

75. Bell RP, Foxe JJ, Ross LA, Garavan H. Intact inhibitory control processes in abstinent drug abusers (I): a functional neuroimaging study in former cocaine addicts. *Neuropharmacology*. 2014;82:143-150. doi:10.1016/j.neuropharm.2013.02.018.

# Where can I get further information about cocaine?

To learn more about cocaine and other drugs of abuse, visit the NIDA website at www.drugabuse.gov or contact *DrugPubs* at 877-NIDA-NIH (877-643-2644; TTY/TDD: 240-645-0228).

## NIDA's website includes:

- Information on drugs of abuse and related health consequences
- NIDA publications, news, and events
- Resources for health care professionals, educators, and patients and families
- Information on NIDA research studies and clinical trials
- Funding information (including program announcements and deadlines)
- International activities
- Links to related websites (access to websites of many other organizations in the field)
- Information in Spanish (en español)

## NIDA websites and webpages

- www.drugabuse.gov
- www.teens.drugabuse.gov
- www.easyread.drugabuse.gov
- www.drugabuse.gov/drugs-abuse/cocaine
- www.researchstudies.drugabuse.gov
- www.irp.drugabuse.gov

## For physician information

- NIDAMED: www.drugabuse.gov/nidamed

## Other websites

Information on cocaine abuse is also available through the following Web site:

- Substance Abuse and Mental Health Services Administration: www.samhsa.gov
- Drug Enforcement Administration: www.dea.gov
- Monitoring the Future: www.monitoringthefuture.org/
- The Partnership at Drug Free.org: www.drugfree.org/drug-guide

This publication is available for your use and may be reproduced **in its entirety** without permission from the NIDA. Citation of the source is appreciated, using the following language: Source: National Institute on Drug Abuse; National Institutes of Health; U.S. Department of Health and Human Services.

www.ingramcontent.com/pod-product-compliance
Lightning Source LLC
Chambersburg PA
CBHW082123220526
45472CB00009B/2280